MW01502913

This Journal
Belongs To:

Made in the
USA
Columbia, SC

81810130R00067